Exploring

Neurodiversity

and

Invisible Disabilities

Exploring Neurodiversity
and
Invisible Disabilities

Authors
Austin Mardon
Lydia C. Rehman, Varun Srikanth, Mehvish Masood,
Adham H. El Sherbini, Mustafa Abbas Zain, Minji Kang,
Natanel Krieksfeld, Daivat Bhavsar

Edited by
Catherine Mardon

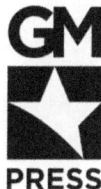

GM
PRESS

Cover Design and typeset by Clare Dalton

Print ISBN 978-1-77889-024-6
Ebook ISBN 978-1-77889-025-3

Golden Meteorite Press
103 11919 82 St NW
Edmonton, AB T5B 2W3
www.goldenmeteoritepress.com

Contents

Chapter 1:
Introducing Neurodiversity

Adham H. El Sherbini

Introduction

In the late 1990s, an Australian sociologist, Judy Singer, introduced
the term neurodiversity to encourage the inclusion of those with
neurological differences (Chapman, 2020). Neurodiversity is best
understood as the neurological distinctions as an aftermath of normal
variability in the human genome. While the definition is broad, autism
spectrum disorder (ASD), attention-deficit/hyperactivity disorder
(ADHD), dyslexia, dyspraxic, and other social anxiety disorders
fall under this umbrella term. While the movement is productive in
achieving its goals, some critics argue that the movement does not
account for difficulties in the quality of life of neurodiverse individuals.
Contrarily, neurodiversity activists typically reckon the term to
represent the inclusion and acceptance of neurodiverse individuals.
These differences in opinions beg the question: How do neurodiverse
individuals cope with their daily lives? To Judy Singer and her fellow
neurodiverse advocates, the solution towards a better quality of life
for neurodiverse individuals lies in accepting neurodiverse-identifying
individuals in our communities, schools, and workplace. However,
to the anti-neurodiversity movement, focus should be prioritized
in the hands of medical research to resolve these differences. This
chapter uncovers the movement's short history, the argumentative and
opposition side, and what we can take away from the term.

Autism Spectrum Disorder

Although the definition varies slightly across professional institutions, autism spectrum disorder (ASD) is best understood as a deviation in brain development that, as a result, influences social interaction and perception (Hodges et al., 2020). Several conditions fall under this umbrella term, including autism, childhood disintegrative disorder (CDD), and Asperger's syndrome. Observation and onset of ASD can be as early as 1-year of age through apparent symptoms, such as difficulty with emotional processing, maintaining eye contact, communication, and non-verbal gestures. While other conditions fall under ASD, the term highlights the variability in symptoms and types of autism, hence the term "spectrum". Researchers have yet to find the underlying sources of the disorder, but the general hypothesis is that ASD is influenced by genetic predispositions and social determinants of health. As a result, risk factors of autism include older parents, siblings diagnosed with ASD, a low birth weight, and the presence of additional genetic conditions. The condition is typically accurately diagnosed at two years of age and screening can be conducted through an evaluation of development and social behavior. Physicians can prescribe certain medications to mediate troublesome symptoms, such as social anxiety and depression, hyperactivity, and difficulty focusing.

Attention Deficit/Hyperactivity Disorder

ADHD presents in childhood, and unlike other children that grow out of being distracted, those with ADHD may encounter the inability to focus throughout their life (Wilens & Spencer, 2010). Common symptoms of ADHD include daydreaming, fidgeting, and excessive talking, however each person's experience with ADHD may be very diverse. To date, three forms of ADHD exist based on the presented symptoms. (1) Predominantly hyperactive-impulsive is a form where most symptoms are centered around hyperactivity. For example, an individual who can not sit for an extended period of time without fidgeting. (2)

Inattentive is when the individual is primarily unable to stay focused and complete a task. (3) This type of ADHD is a combination of both subtypes. Compared to ASD, there is no solidified cause of ADHD, but researchers believe that both genetics and social factors could influence its onset. Those diagnosed with ADHD may have exposure to toxic substances, like alcohol or tobacco during pregnancy and have possible injuries to the brain. The prevalence of ADHD within the population hovers around 5%.

Dyslexia and Other Neurodiverse Conditions

Similarly, dyslexia is a learning-centric disorder that is otherwise known as a reading disability (Snowling et al., 2020). It influences aspects of the brain in charge of language, making it difficult to decode pieces of literature into speech sounds. Dyslexia is one of the neurodivergent conditions where emotional and social support is necessary as its severity is entirely dependent on that. One who is dyslexic but is provided with consistent support throughout their education can succeed, as seen in the case of Albert Einstein, Walt Disney, and John F. Kennedy (Famous Dyslexics & Celebrities | Helen Arkell Dyslexia Centre, 2013). However, since the students may face differences in the phonological aspects of language processing, pupils with dyslexia can undergo different methods of preferred learning within the classroom. Although difficult to measure, the prevalence of dyslexia lingers at around 10% of the total population. Therefore, in countries where education is not personalized, this condition can become more visible..

Similarly, dyspraxia, also called developmental coordination disorder, is a condition that affects one's coordination, including balance, motor operation, or playing sports (Gibbs et al., 2007). Typically, a diagnosis of dyspraxia is conducted by physiotherapists or occupational therapists through the conduction of a number of tests. To add, those with dyspraxia are also prone to additional neurodiverse conditions, including autism, ADHD, dyslexia, and dyscalculia (differences in doing math). Although this condition can affect one's quality of life, there are a number of ways to improve one's coordination, such as exercise, practice, and improving organization. Finally, although the focal conditions of neurodiversity have been highlighted, there remains additional conditions that fall under the term (dysgraphia, Meares-Irlen syndrome, Tourette's syndrome, and obsessive compulsive disorder (OCD)).

A word, mission, and movement

The perception of neurodiversity varies between individuals. To some, it's a term to collect similar conditions; to others, it is a mission recognizing neurological conditions; and to Judy Singer and fellow advocates, neurodiversity is a movement to provide inclusion and acceptance to these individuals. As their recognition of these conditions is relatively new, it begs the question of how we should interpret neurodiverse disorders. For example, many individuals with ASD have special abilities that would otherwise not be observed in non-ASD individuals. This raises a debate on how these skills should be utilized. Regardless of belief or opinion, fundamental aspects of neurodiversity are worth understanding and respecting. For one, this movement wishes to provide a more inclusive space for those with neurological disabilities, as they are no less of a person than anyone else (Armstrong, 2015). Where the sides typically differ is in the classifications of the conditions and human variations in the brain. On the first point, some neurodiverse individuals would classify neurodiverse conditions as differences rather than disabilities. Contrarily, those not in favor of the term would consider these conditions as disabilities in the social standard. On a more important note, regardless of the overarching headline, difference or disability, all spaces (ie. work, public, educational) should ensure they are inclusive to meet the needs of people who may not think or act neurotypical.

Regarding vital variability, those supporting the neurodiverse system believe that all humans live with vital variations in neurological development. While true, others argue that there are set out markers for these disorders, and they are not simply a natural variation in the human mind. Although these opinions are distinct, it is necessary to find a middle ground as higher-level beliefs will ultimately determine the translation of policy changes into effect.

Where should attention be prioritized?

Many neurodiverse advocates believe that the underlying conditions should not be extinguished from society, as they are an essential element of these humans. Instead, living and managing neurodivergence lies in the communities to provide an accommodating space for these individuals, as is provided for all humans. Although such arrangements vary per condition, such changes are expected to be implemented in workplaces, communities, schools, and public settings. Some of these can include headphones to prevent auditory overstimulation and implementing methods in communities to ensure equality across all neurodiverse individuals. Moreover, the addition of neurodiverse individuals in the workplace can benefit them as they can be exceptionally skilled in specific job tasks. With this solution of equality, individuals, regardless of neurological development are equal in opportunities. While some may argue that such focus ignores the challenges these individuals suffer, it's important to remember that the clinical research has been unproductive. Society is not naturally designed to support the needs of neurodiverse peoples, due to a lack of understanding and ignorance. However, despite this, being able to provide awareness, and understanding within systems to rethink the way spaces are designed ensure inclusivity of neurodivergence and invisible disabilities is where attention should be prioritized.

Conclusion

Neurodiversity is more than just an umbrella term to cover conditions that undergo neurological differences. It is a movement to embrace the conditions and provide a degree of treatment that would otherwise be deemed equal if provided to non-neurodiverse individuals. Like all other movements, there remains an opposition side that believes these conditions should be placed in a more negative light rather than being acknowledged as natural variations in human development. However, regardless of one's opinion, the lack of research should prompt a society that is more inclusive of neurodiverse individuals and provides them with the opportunity to accomplish just as much as their non-neurodiverse counterparts.

References

Chapman, R. (2020). Defining neurodiversity for research and practice. Neurodiversity Studies, 218–220. https://doi.org/10.4324/9780429322297-21

Hodges, H., Fealko, C., & Soares, N. (2020). Autism spectrum disorder: definition, epidemiology, causes, and clinical evaluation. Translational Pediatrics, 9(S1), S55–S65. https://doi.org/10.21037/tp.2019.09.09

Wilens, T. E., & Spencer, T. J. (2010). Understanding Attention-Deficit/ Hyperactivity Disorder from Childhood to Adulthood. Postgraduate Medicine, 122(5), 97–109. https://doi.org/10.3810/pgm.2010.09.2206

Snowling, M. J., Hulme, C., & Nation, K. (2020). Defining and understanding dyslexia: past, present and future. Oxford Review of Education, 46(4), 501–513. https://doi.org/10.1080/03054985.2020.1765756

Famous Dyslexics & Celebrities | Helen Arkell Dyslexia Centre. (2013). Helenarkell.org.uk. https://www.helenarkell.org.uk/about-dyslexia/famous-dyslexics.php

Gibbs, J., Appleton, J., & Appleton, R. (2007). Dyspraxia or developmental coordination disorder? Unravelling the enigma. Archives of Disease in Childhood, 92(6), 534–539. https://doi.org/10.1136/adc.2005.088054

Armstrong, T. (2015). The Myth of the Normal Brain: Embracing Neurodiversity. AMA Journal of Ethics, 17(4), 348–352. https://doi.org/10.1001/journalofethics.2015.17.4.msoc1-1504

Chapter 2: An Overview of Mental Health Disorders

Mehvish Masood*, HBMSc (c)

A variety of mental health disabilities impact a large amount of the world's population. These tend to be anxiety, major depression, bipolar disorders, schizophrenia, and borderline personality disorder. Understanding these disorders is important in reducing the stigma and helping those in question. This chapter will give a brief overview of each of these disorders, along with how diagnosis criteria occur, causes, and treatment plans.

Anxiety

Anxiety disorders are a range of conditions that include generalized anxiety disorder (GAD), social anxiety disorder, specific phobias, panic disorders, and more. It is considered the most prevalent psychiatric disorder, with women being more likely than men to receive a diagnosis for the disorder (Bandelow et al., 2017). The onset of anxiety disorders depends on the condition. For example, specific phobias start during childhood, while GAD may start later in life (Bandelow et al., 2017). The cause or etiology of anxiety disorders are often complex and are not entirely understood. Currently, it is thought that environmental and genetic factors have contributed to some level. Life events between childhood and adolescence play a significant role in environmental factors. For example, some experiences include with sexual or physical violence; separation from family; and physical illness (Deckert, 2009). That said, twin and family studies have revealed an exciting role in genetics. Association and linkage studies have identified locations on chromosomes, for example, 13q and 22q, that are relevant to anxiety disorders (Deckert, 2009). Research has already shown, however, that genetics and the environment contribute to some but not all percent of the variance. Scientists are still looking into the complex and multi-faceted factors (Deckert, 2009).

Similar to other mental health disorders, anxiety disorders are defined within categories. The IDC-10 and DSM-5 are classification systems commonly used in psychology and include anxiety disorder classification guidelines (Deckert, 2009). Regardless, diagnosing these disorders requires a careful inspection of the individual. Much care is put into ensuring that it is not another health condition associated with physiologic changes within the body. This can include epilepsies and hyperthecosis. Therefore, electrocardiograms, routine blood tests, and electroencephalograms must be performed before diagnosis (Deckert, 2009). Other steps may be necessary following before making a concrete diagnosis. On top of this, anxiety can also be a symptom of other mental health disorders, so a careful eye must be used for diagnosis (Deckert, 2009).

There are several forms of treatment for anxiety disorders, many of which must be individualized for the person in question for the best results. Psychotherapy, which may involve supportive talks and attention to emotional problems associated with the disorder, is essential for patients (Bandelow et al., 2017). Cognitive behavioral therapy, specifically, has shown to be highly effective in various trials and is considered a prevalent treatment form(Bandelow et al., 2017). However, specific drug types can also help with specific anxiety disorders.

Efficacy for GAD, social anxiety disorder, and panic disorder has been shown in several studies, whereas there are very few studies on drug treatments for specific phobias (Bandelow et al., 2017).

Major Depression

Major depression, also known as clinical depression, is a mental health disorder associated with persistent loss of interest and feelings of sadness. Notably, depression is not a weakness that people can simply eliminate. Long-term treatment often involves psychotherapy and medications, if not both ("Depression (major depressive disorder)," 2018). Many symptoms are associated with depression. They include feelings of sadness, emptiness, and hopelessness. Anxiety and restlessness with recurring suicidal thoughts are also symptoms of depression. These symptoms often manifest to a point where day-to-day activities such as social activities, school, and work may be affected. Notably, the symptoms present in adults are very similar to children and teens, with slight differences. For example, in teens, symptoms may include poor performance in school, use of drugs or alcohol, and avoidance of social interaction. Furthermore, depression is not a normal part of growing older and often is undiagnosed because older adults may be less likely to seek help. Symptoms of depression in older adults may manifest as memory difficulties, pain, fatigue, or loss of appetite that is not caused by a medical condition or medication ("Depression (major depressive disorder)," 2018).

As with other mental health disorders, the cause of depression is multifaceted and extremely complex. It may involve physical differences in the shape of people's brains ("Depression (major depressive disorder)," 2018). Alternatively, it may have to do with brain chemistry. The function and impact of neurotransmitters, which are essentially the chemical messengers in the brain, are different in depressed patients. These changes may be involved with maintaining mood stability and can play a significant role in depression ("Depression (major depressive disorder)," 2018). Aside from the brain, hormones may play a role in depression. Hormones are messengers sent in the bloodstream to deliver "signals" to other body parts to perform specific functions. They are often released in response to stimuli such as low blood sugar. Hormone levels change after pregnancy and menopause, which may be associated with depression ("Depression (major depressive disorder)," 2018). Further, depression can be partly inherited. Those with blood relatives with the condition are more likely to have it, suggesting a genetic linkage. Research is currently looking into the specific genes associated with depression ("Depression (major depressive disorder)," 2018).

Bipolar Disorders

Fluctuations in energy and mood state characterize bipolar disorders. This disorder affects more than 1% of the world's population and is prevalent across ethnic groups and cultures (Grande et al., 2015). This disorder is a lifelong illness that occurs episodically and significantly impact the quality of life. Diagnosis of bipolar disorders is often difficult because the symptoms are very similar to depression, and no distinctive biological markersdefine bipolar disorders (Grande et al., 2015). Further research looks into this condition to find more information about the diagnosis. Treatment for bipolar disorder occurs after diagnosis and involves medications at times. For example, mood stabilizers like lithium and antipsychotics like haloperidol may be used (Grande et al., 2015).

There are several types of bipolar disorders based on the DSM-5 system of mental illness diagnosis (Grande et al., 2015). The types vary depending on the type of episode. To explain this, manic must be defined. Manic or hypomanic episodes are states of elevated moods. Individuals experiencing these episodes have elevated cognitive function and persist for a finite time: 4 consecutive days for hypomanic episodes and one week for manic episodes (Grande et al., 2015). With that being said, we will discuss the most common types of bipolar disorders. Bipolar I disorder occurs when there must be one manic episode, with major depressive episodes being typical but not necessary for diagnosis. Bipolar II disorder has at least one hypomanic and one major depressive episode. Cyclothymic disorders are hypomanic and depressive periods that do not fulfill hypomania or major depression criteria, respectively, for at least two years. Bipolar disorders that do not meet the criteria for the three previously mentioned types of bipolar disorders because of insufficient duration or severity are classified as other specified bipolar and related disorders (Grande et al., 2015).

Schizophrenia

Schizophrenia is a complex disorder that has a significant effect on those impacted. It is characterized by delusions, hallucinations, disorganized speech, and impaired cognitive ability. More specifically, the symptoms associated with schizophrenia are categorized into positive and negative symptoms. Positive symptoms are associated with behavioral changes, whereas negative symptoms are associated with a loss of consciousness of the world or deficits (Patel et al., 2014). The diagnostic criterion for schizophrenia involves the following five symptoms: (1)Delusions, (2)Hallucinations, (3)Disorganized Speech, (4)Grossly disorganized or catatonic behavior, and (5) negative symptoms. Individuals must present two or more of the five symptoms listed for three months or longer to be diagnosed. In addition, they must present one of the initial three listed symptoms (delusions, hallucinations, disorganized speech) (McCutcheon et al., 2020). On top of this, impairments of a major area of function for a substantial period since onset and signs of the disorder must last for at least six months. Notably, this is the primary criterion, with additional details to consider for diagnosis (McCutcheon et al., 2020).

Borderline Personality Disorder

A borderline personality disorder is a complex mental health condition associated with pervasive patterns of instability in impulse control, interpersonal relationships, self-image, and more. It impacts 1-2% of the general population and is associated with high suicide rates (Lieb et al., 2004). Similar to other disorders, the cause of borderline personality disorder is complex. Adverse childhood experiences are thought to play a role, which includes neglect and abuse at a young age. However, genetics also is thought to have an impact (Lieb et al., 2004). According to the DSM-5, there are four criteria patients must satisfy to be considered for borderline personality disorder (Lieb et al., 2004). The first is an affective disturbance, which involves having extreme moods of rage, sorrow, shame, terror, and loneliness. In addition, these individuals have extreme mood reactivity, where they can change moods from one state to another with great rapidness and fluidity. The second and third criteria are disturbed cognition and impulsivity, respectively. The last is unstable relationships, which may manifest as an intense fear of abandonment or a pattern of intense interpersonal relationships (Lieb et al., 2004). If an individual expresses all four of these criteria, they are considered to have a borderline personality disorder. Notably, those with borderline personality disorder also meet the criteria for other illnesses –for example, post-traumatic stress disorder, major depression, and more (Lieb et al., 2004).

Conclusion

This chapter went over the common mental health disorders that many individuals exhibit. First, anxiety disorders pertain to various conditions, including generalized anxiety disorder, specific phobias and more. Next, major depression is a condition that is often associated with persistent feelings of loss and sadness. Alternatively, bipolar disorders are identified by fluctuating moods and states. Moreover, schizophrenia is characterized by hallucinations, delusions, and changes in speech. Last, a bipolar personality disorder is related to pervasive patterns related to impulse control, self-image, and more. The DSM-5 aids with setting the guidelines for these conditions and is an important part of mental health conditions and research. Overall, understanding these various mental health disorders is important in reducing stigma and helping individuals. For this reason, the increased research and understanding of such subjects is fascinating and will help make the world a better place.

References

Bandelow, B., Michaelis, S., & Wedekind, D. (2017). Treatment of anxiety disorders. Dialogues in clinical neuroscience, 19(2), 93–107. https://doi. org/10.31887/DCNS.2017.19.2/bbandelow

Deckert. (2009). Anxiety disorders: causes, diagnosis and treatment. Acta Neuropsychiatrica, 21(S2), 9–10. https://doi.org/10.1017/S0924270800032592

Grande, Berk, M., Birmaher, B., & Vieta, E. (2015). Bipolar disorder. The Lancet (British Edition), 387(10027), 1561–1572. https://doi.org/10.1016/S0140-6736(15)00241-X

Lieb, K., Zanarini, M. C., Schmahl, C., Linehan, M. M., & Bohus, M. (2004). Borderline personality disorder. Lancet (London, England), 364(9432), 453–461. https://doi.org/10.1016/S0140-6736(04)16770-6

Mayo Foundation for Medical Education and Research. (2018, February 3). Depression (major depressive disorder). Mayo Clinic. Retrieved July 30, 2022, from https://www.mayoclinic.org/diseases-conditions/depression/symptoms-causes/syc-20356007

McCutcheon, R. A., Reis Marques, T., & Howes, O. D. (2020). Schizophrenia-An Overview. JAMA psychiatry, 77(2), 201–210. https://doi.org/10.1001/jamapsychiatry.2019.3360

Patel, K. R., Cherian, J., Gohil, K., & Atkinson, D. (2014). Schizophrenia: overview and treatment options. P & T : a peer-reviewed journal for formulary management, 39(9), 638–645.

Chapter 3: Overview of Attention-Deficit/Hyperactivity Disorder

Varun Srikanth* HBHSc

Introduction

Attention-deficit/hyperactivity disorder (ADHD) is defined as a "persistent pattern of inattention and/or hyperactivity-impulsivity that interferes with functioning or development" (CDC, n.d.; American Psychiatric Association [APA], 2013). Our understanding of ADHD has gradually evolved; historically, there were two dominant perspectives. Either it was considered an entirely neuropathological condition resulting from certain genetic predispositions and the influence of one's physical environment; or simply a human psychological variant (Berri & Al-Hroub, 2016). Today, ADHD is understood as a "developmental, neurobiological condition defined by the presence of severe and pervasive symptoms of inattention, hyperactivity, and impulsivity" (Berri & Al-Hroub, 2016).

The global prevalence of ADHD is estimated to be between two and seven percent, with an average of 5%. According to several population-based surveys, the prevalence of ADHD in children is five percent and two-and-a-half percent in adults (Mohammadi et al., 2021). While the exact etiological mechanisms are unclear, it is understood to be a combination of genetic, neurological, and environmental facts. In addition, sex-based studies demonstrate that ADHD is two to three times more common in males than females, and age-based explorations show

that its prevalence increases up to the age of nine and subsequently
decreases in both genders (Erskine, 2013; Mohammadi et al., 2021;
Sayal, 2018). With these ideas in mind, this chapter aims to provide
an overview of ADHD, how it is diagnosed, and the current treatment
options available to patients and their families.

Causes of ADHD

Overview

The etiological mechanisms of ADHD are undetermined; however, its
causes are multifactorial and involve a nuanced relationship between
several genetic and environmental factors (Faraone et al., 2021). Many
studies have established that genes and their relationship with the
environment play a profound role in the etiology of ADHD, albeit a
more substantial influence from genetic abnormalities. Interestingly,
the environmental risks for ADHD are found to exert their effects
early in one's development—during the fetal or early postnatal period
specifically. In rare cases, ADHD-like symptoms can emerge from
extreme early-life events or irregularities, including a single genetic
abnormality, traumatic brain injury, and severe deprivation. It is
important to note that while the presence of these early-life events
or genetic irregularities is critical in understanding the causes of
ADHD, they are not substantial enough to make a confident diagnosis.
The following section aims to delineate recent genetic insights and
environmental risk factors for ADHD.

Genetic Insights

ADHD has one of the highest inheritance rates among
neurodevelopmental disorders—ranging from 54% to more than 70%
of cases (Kian et al., 2022). One study investigated the severity of
ADHD between offspring of parents with ADHD and parents without;
it was found that offspring of the former group were more likely to

develop severe forms of the disorder (Kian et al., 2022; Takeda, 2010). While the results did not indicate an interdependent influence of biparental ADHD, maternal and paternal ADHD status seems to have differing effects on ADHD symptoms in offspring (Kian et al., 2022; Takeda, 2010). In addition, some studies have investigated the genome of children and adults with ADHD; interestingly, one study found that the children shared certain genetic variant forms pertaining to certain oxidative stress proteins, DISC1, DBH, DDC, microRNA, and adiponectin genes (Kian et al., 2022; Bonvicini, 2018). Simply put, the genes mentioned above play several different roles, from regulating neural development and brain maturation to providing the genetic instructions for manufacturing crucial enzymes involved in neural functioning (Bonvicini, 2018).

There is also a significant association between various patterns of methylation in dopaminergic and serotonergic genes and the severity of the behavioural phenotype of ADHD children (Kian et al., 2022). DNA methylation is a process of adding a methyl group—a chemical structure that contains one carbon and three hydrogen atoms—to different compounds in our bodies (Moore, 2013). This process is essential because it ensures the optimal functioning of compounds, like enzymes and hormones, and facilitates the creation of other required compounds in our body (Moore, 2013). In the context of ADHD, one study found that the increased methylation of the promoter region of the serotonin-transporter gene (5-HTT) was associated with more severe ADHD symptoms (Park et al., 2015). The gene promoter region is a DNA sequence that indicates the gene's starting point and acts as a landmark for its duplication (Park et al., 2015). However, increased promoter region methylation has been shown to reduce gene expression, meaning that methylation of the 5-HTT gene would result in lower levels of serotonin—a mood stabilizing neurotransmitter—in the synaptic cleft (Park et al., 2015). Studies show that chronically low serotonin levels at this junction where neurons communicate may trigger ADHD symptoms (Park et al., 2015). Like this, many associations with various gene variants have been investigated, but further studies are needed to refine our understanding (Kian et al., 2022).

Environmental Risk Factors

Prenatal environmental risk factors don't contribute to ADHD symptoms to the same degree as genetic risk factors; however, their influence on ADHD onset has been investigated extensively (Kian et al., 2022). Importantly, the literature on prenatal environmental risk factors lacks consistency because a single risk factor cannot induce ADHD symptoms; instead, it's the combination of these risk factors that has a compounding effect. Despite this inconsistency, it is known that the risk factors for ADHD symptoms can be categorized: symptoms of inattentiveness are typically influenced by psychosocial risk factors, and hyperactive-impulsive symptoms are more likely to be induced by biological risk factors. Recent studies have demonstrated nine significant associations between prenatal environmental risk factors and ADHD. The most profound were maternal smoking, pre-pregnancy obesity, and acetaminophen use during pregnancy.

It is known that exposure to smoking during pregnancy has many deleterious effects on fetal development (Kian et al., 2022). Maternal smoking increases the risk of ADHD symptoms in offspring by 2.7-fold, and there is a 2-fold greater risk of offspring developing ADHD in mothers who have used or have been exposed to tobacco during pregnancy. While maternal and paternal smoking is associated with ADHD in offspring, maternal smoking has a more significant influence. Cigarette smoking negatively affects embryonic development as it can interfere with placental functioning, disrupt fetal blood flow, and deprive the fetus of oxygen and essential nutrients for growth and development. Studies have also found the risk of ADHD differs in children of mothers who are heavy and light smokers. Expectedly, mothers who are heavy

smokers during pregnancy—that is, more than ten cigarettes per day—
had ADHD children with significantly higher psychosocial stress than
unaffected children.

Exposure to certain dietary components also influences ADHD
pathogenesis, like alcohol (Kian et al., 2022). During fetal development,
the developing brain is susceptible to alcohol; exposure to alcohol
during this period can disrupt neurodevelopment—especially in
the cerebellum, which is involved in physical movement and motor
skills— and increase the likelihood of anomalies arising (Kian et
al., 2022). Evidence of heavy metal exposure during pregnancy and
ADHD has also been observed in the literature (Banerjee et al., 2007).
For instance, people of New Zealand and the Faroe Islands are more
likely to consume mercury-contaminated fish. Expectant mothers in
these regions, who consumed the contaminated fish, had offspring with
higher rates of memory disruption, inattention, lower IQ compared
to other children, and impaired motor skills (Banerjee et al., 2007).
Similarly, neurodevelopment is also affected in the offspring of mothers
with poor diets. Dietary components like long-chain polyunsaturated
fatty acids and minerals, such as zinc and magnesium, are crucial in
the normal development of the fetal brain (Kian et al., 2022). Mothers
who are chronically deficient in polyunsaturated omega-3 fatty acids—
particularly DHA—had children with an increased risk of ADHD
(Kian et al., 2022).

Consumption of certain drugs during pregnancy also seems to increase
the risk of ADHD onset in offspring; namely, acetaminophen use
was associated with higher rates of ADHD in children (Kian et al.,
2022). While the mechanisms are unclear, one study suggested that
acetaminophen interferes with endogenous hormones and signaling
pathways during fetal development (Masarwa et al., 2018). It is also
important to note that the longer duration of acetaminophen use is
associated with more severe ADHD symptoms, whereas short-term

use negatively correlates with ADHD in the offspring (Kian et al., 2022; Ystrom et al., 2017). However, consumption of drugs like anti-depressants, anti-seizure medications, and prenatal antibiotics during pregnancy had inconsistent results in the literature; a lack of conclusive evidence is due to the heterogeneity of the study results and potentially unarticulated confounding factors (Kian et al., 2022).

ADHD Diagnosis

Overview

A licensed clinician must diagnose ADHD, typically in young patients four years or older (Felt et al., 2014; CAMH, n.d.). The literature observes a higher prevalence of ADHD in males than females; however, a general rule of thumb is that the inattentive phenotype is associated with females. Therefore, parents and guardians, friends, and others involved in the patient's life should be watchful for the above indicators and address concerns about behavioral differences by seeking professional medical guidance from a licensed physician or a mental health specialist. While the evaluation of ADHD is unstandardized, diagnostic criteria presented in the fifth edition of the Diagnostic and Statistical Manual of Mental Disorders (DSM) provide meaningful direction in understanding patients' symptomatology.

The DSM classifies ADHD into three clinical presentations: predominantly inattentive, predominantly hyperactive-impulsive, and a combined phenotype (CDC, n.d.; APA, 2013). As the name suggests, the predominantly inattentive presentation of symptoms is when the patient is more inattentive than hyperactive-impulsive (Felt et al., 2014). Typically, this means the patient is often distracted, has poor organizational skills, and has difficulty completing tasks and following through with objectives (Felt et al., 2014). In contrast, the predominantly hyperactive-impulsive presentation describes a patient presenting more symptoms of this behavioral phenotype than inattentiveness (Felt et al., 2014). Common indicators of this subtype include fidgetiness, a tendency to interrupt others during conversations or tasks, and overly active behavior (Felt et al., 2014). Finally, the combined subtype is when the patient's symptoms fit both criteria. A fundamental diagnostic criterion for patients with ADHD symptoms is that their symptoms should have persisted for at least six months before their examination (Felt et al., 2014). Moreover, it is important to note that these symptoms can change over time; as a result, their presentation and diagnosis may evolve parallelly (CAMH, n.d.).

In general, diagnosing ADHD includes reviewing the patient's medical history to delineate birth history, early developmental progressions, medications, and concurrent psychological and physical evaluations (Felt et al., 2014; Subcommittee on Attention-Deficit/ Hyperactivity Disorder, Steering Committee on Quality Improvement and Management, 2011). Additionally, the patient's physician or mental health professional will conduct interviews to understand the reporting of the patient's ADHD symptoms across multiple contexts: parent/caregiver report of symptoms and other medical conditions, a school/community report of the patient's symptoms outside of a home environment, and a patient's report of their own symptoms and how it's affecting their life. Typically, school-related reporting also involves a summary of the patient's academic performance, like absenteeism and grade retention. Finally, behavioral ratings from validated ADHD screening tools from the aforementioned contexts also contribute to the overall assessment.

ADHD Evaluation

In preschool-aged children—below the age of four years—ADHD cannot be reliably diagnosed; even at four and five years of age, it is difficult to gauge whether presenting behaviour is aligned with expected behaviour for this age cohort (Felt et al., 2014). Despite this challenge, validated behavioural rating scales can improve diagnostic confidence. For example, ACTeRS Rating Scale, validated for children in kindergarten to eighth grade, is assessed in tandem with a parent and teacher report. Another is the Attention Deficit Disorder Evaluation Scale, fourth edition, which—also used in tandem with a parent and teacher report—assesses patients aged four to eighteen.

In older children, ADHD symptoms typically arise in their elementary schooling years (Felt et al., 2014). Patients with a predominantly hyperactive-impulsive or combined subtype may present symptoms deemed problematic by teachers or parents before those with the predominantly inattentive subtype. Moreover, the former patient population may only present non-trivial symptoms with increased academic requirements that accompany higher grade levels, like the fourth or fifth grade. Therefore, an important consideration when evaluating older children is the presence of comorbidities common with ADHD diagnoses. In fact, the literature states that one-third of ADHD patients have comorbidity; these include a comorbid learning disorder, sleep-related issues like sleep apnea, adenotonsillar hypertrophy, neuromuscular abnormalities, and even obesity. Interestingly, some comorbidities, like sleep problems, can significantly impact daytime functioning and may even mimic ADHD symptomatology.

New onset of ADHD symptoms in adolescents—beyond twelve years—is less common but possible with greater academic demands or if subtle signs had gone unnoticed when they were younger (Felt et al., 2014). Like older children, comorbid learning disabilities, mental health conditions, and more nuanced issues like substance abuse should be considered during diagnosis due to overlapping presentations. The literature suggests that ADHD evaluation in this patient population should be informed by the insights provided by at least two teachers who know the patient well and potentially another supervisory adult, like a coach. Moreover, at this age, self-report behavioral screening tools are also available; despite potential reliability concerns, it is generally accepted that these tools complement the parent and teacher scales and aid in understanding the patient's internalized states.

ADHD evaluation in adults is more challenging than in children due to a lack of clarity in the diagnostic criteria. Moreover, the manifestations of ADHD symptoms differ throughout one's life, albeit the underlying symptoms are similar in both children and adults (Adler et al., 2009). One study found that primary care physicians were not confident in diagnosing ADHD in their adult patients and were more likely to defer their diagnosis to a mental health specialist (Adler et al., 2009). Despite these challenges, the Canadian ADHD Research Alliance has developed the Canadian ADHD Practice Guidelines—endorsed by the Centre for Addiction and Mental Health (CAMH)—which can aid primary care physicians in gathering a more nuanced understanding of their patient's experiences (Canadian ADHD Resource Alliance [CADDRA], n.d.). Using an evidence-based approach, these guidelines were developed and codified by a multidisciplinary team of medical and health professionals from Canada and the United States (CADDRA, n.d.). They outline ADHD diagnosis, assessment, and treatment across a patient's lifespan; provide expert consensus when evidence is lacking; offer clinical advice; provide screening tools for patients and their caregivers (CADDRA, n.d.). Although the aforementioned tools and guidelines may facilitate a diagnosis, none can confidently make one or provide a threshold marker for a patient's cognitive status (CAMH, n.d.).

ADHD Treatment

Overview

The primary objective of ADHD treatment is to reduce the severity of the patient's symptoms, improve functional performance, and subdue persistent behavioral hurdles (Felt et al., 2014). Physicians and mental health specialists should also provide ADHD-specific education and resources to equip parents and families with the tools to understand how they can best support their children. Moreover, parents can ask their child's school and school district board to provide accommodation as outlined by regulation. School support can come in many forms and is tailored to the child's needs, which are iterated in an individualized education plan (IEP). These peripheral supports are essential in addition to the patient's therapeutic prescriptions.

Generally speaking, children under six years with ADHD should begin behavioral therapy (Felt et al., 2014). Medications for this age cohort should only be considered if symptoms are moderate to severe and the patient is unresponsive to behavioral therapy. The opposite is recommended for patients older than six; if these patients are less responsive to pharmaceutical therapies, behavioral therapy is an excellent complement to their treatment plan.

Non-pharmacological Therapies

Psychological and behavioral interventions are highly effective in ADHD treatment and management (Hodgson et al., 2014). However, behavioral therapies' lack of validation and standardization is one drawback. Furthermore, recent meta-analyses lack a comprehensive review of the interventions and their comparative efficacies. Nevertheless, seven primary behavioral therapies have shown promise, and the following section will provide an overview of these therapies.

The behavioral modification approach involves principles of learning theory and operant conditioning (Hodgson et al., 2014). It utilizes positive and negative reinforcement techniques to improve the child's behavior. Neurofeedback is a newer non-pharmacological therapy for ADHD and has been shown in the literature to be promising. Patients are trained to control particular brainwave patterns using electroencephalographic technology, which increases beta activity while decreasing theta activity. The effect of this therapy is targeted at improving attention and concentration, which by extension, is a physiological means of developing self-control. Multimodal psychosocial treatment integrates individual psychological interventions to target symptoms across multiple functional domains, like behavioral, neuropsychological, and academic areas. School-based psychological programming integrates principles of behavior modification and cognitive-behavior modification techniques but applies them in a classroom setting to help teachers and students gain control of behavior. As the name suggests, working memory training aims to strengthen and train working memory—limited capacity, temporary memory used to perform cognitive tasks. This technique uses a computerized task specific to the person's skill level and becomes more difficult as the training progresses. Parent training involves teaching parents to use strategies with particular therapeutic goals in mind to gain greater control of their children's behavior; simultaneously, the children are taught a set of skills to use at home to improve their behavior. Finally, self-monitoring relies on self-regulation by virtue of completing a checklist of the behaviors one has engaged in over time.

Pharmacological Treatments

Stimulant medication is widely used for ADHD due to higher response rates than psychological and non-pharmacological interventions (Felt et al., 2014). The most effective and safe pharmacological treatments are psychostimulants, like methylphenidate, dextroamphetamine, and mixed amphetamine salts, like dextroamphetamine/amphetamine. In national guidelines and reviews, the aforementioned medications are the first choice. Other treatments like atomoxetine and alpha-2 receptor agonists, like clonidine, are efficacious but less effective than psychostimulants. Moreover, they are not the first pharmacological treatment choice because they lack many supporting studies. Other medications like antidepressants, atypical antipsychotics, and mood stabilizers can also be prescribed upon the clinicians' prerogative. Importantly, these medications are not approved by the United States Food and Drug Administration for treating ADHD.

Sometimes PCPs, parents, and children don't want to take stimulant medications (Hodgson et al., 2014). Moreover, it cannot always be prescribed confidently due to its risks, especially when the patient has associated comorbidities. In addition, the long-term effects of stimulant medications are yet to be elucidated, and there is a potential for unintended adverse effects. Moreover, the child may also need to take multiple doses daily, which is inconvenient and a common deterrent for parents and caregivers. Common side effects include nausea, weight loss, insomnia, decreased energy, muscle tension, and, although infrequent, sudden death due to cardiovascular problems. Therefore, clinicians also recommend pursuing a combined approach for optimal symptom reduction and improvement. However, since there is a constant need to further develop and evaluate psychological intervention efficacy in ADHD, stimulant medications are still considered the more productive approach.

References

Adler, L., Shaw, D., Sitt, D., Maya, E., & Morrill, M. (2009). Issues in the Diagnosis and Treatment of Adult ADHD by Primary Care Physicians. Primary Psychiatry, 16.

Banerjee, E., & Nandagopal, K. (2015). Does serotonin deficit mediate susceptibility to ADHD? Neurochemistry International, 82, 52–68. https://doi.org/10.1016/j.neuint.2015.02.001

Banerjee, T. D., Middleton, F., & Faraone, S. V. (2007). Environmental risk factors for attention-deficit hyperactivity disorder. Acta Paediatrica, 96(9), 1269–1274. https://doi.org/10.1111/j.1651-2227.2007.00430.x

Berri, H. M., & Al-Hroub, A. (2016). Introduction to ADHD. In H. M. Berri & A. Al-Hroub (Eds.), ADHD in Lebanese Schools: Diagnosis, Assessment, and Treatment (pp. 1–6). Springer International Publishing. https://doi.org/10.1007/978-3-319-28700-3_1

Bonvicini, C., Faraone, S. V., & Scassellati, C. (2018). Common and specific genes and peripheral biomarkers in children and adults with attention-deficit/hyperactivity disorder. The World Journal of Biological Psychiatry, 19(2), 80–100. https://doi.org/10.1080/15622975.2017.1282175

CADDRA. (n.d.). Download Guidelines. Retrieved August 11, 2022, from https://www.caddra.ca/download-guidelines/

CAMH. (n.d.) Adult ADHD: Screening and Assessment. Retrieved August 11, 2022, from https://www.camh.ca/en/professionals/treating-conditions-and-disorders/adult-adhd/adult-adhd---screening-and-assessment

CDC. (n.d.). Symptoms and Diagnosis of ADHD. Retrieved August 11, 2022, from https://www.cdc.gov/ncbddd/adhd/diagnosis.html

Erskine, H. E., Ferrari, A. J., Nelson, P., Polanczyk, G. V., Flaxman, A. D., Vos, T., Whiteford, H. A., & Scott, J. G. (2013). Research Review: Epidemiological modelling of attention-deficit/hyperactivity disorder and conduct disorder for the Global Burden of Disease Study 2010. Journal of Child Psychology and Psychiatry, 54(12), 1263–1274. https://doi.org/10.1111/jcpp.12144

Faraone, S. V., Banaschewski, T., Coghill, D., Zheng, Y., Biederman, J., Bellgrove, M. A., Newcorn, J. H., Gignac, M., Al Saud, N. M., Manor, I., Rohde, L. A., Yang, L., Cortese, S., Almagor, D., Stein, M. A., Albatti, T. H., Aljoudi, H. F., Alqahtani, M. M. J., Asherson, P., … Wang, Y. (2021). The World Federation of ADHD International Consensus Statement: 208 Evidence-based conclusions about the disorder. Neuroscience & Biobehavioral Reviews, 128, 789–818. https://doi.org/10.1016/j.neubiorev.2021.01.022

Felt, B. T., & Biermann, B. (2014). Diagnosis and Management of ADHD In Children. 90(7), 9.

Hodgson, K., Hutchinson, A. D., & Denson, L. (2014). Nonpharmacological Treatments for ADHD: A Meta-Analytic Review. Journal of Attention Disorders, 18(4), 275–282. https://doi.org/10.1177/1087054712444732

Kian, N., Samieefar, N., & Rezaei, N. (2022). Prenatal risk factors and genetic causes of ADHD in children. World Journal of Pediatrics, 18(5), 308–319. https://doi.org/10.1007/s12519-022-00524-6

Masarwa, R., Levine, H., Gorelik, E., Reif, S., Perlman, A., & Matok, I. (2018). Prenatal Exposure to Acetaminophen and Risk for Attention Deficit Hyperactivity Disorder and Autistic Spectrum Disorder: A Systematic Review, Meta-Analysis, and Meta-Regression Analysis of Cohort Studies. American Journal of Epidemiology, 187(8), 1817–1827. https://doi.org/10.1093/aje/kwy086

Mohammadi, M.-R., Zarafshan, H., Khaleghi, A., Ahmadi, N., Hooshyari, Z., Mostafavi, S.-A., Ahmadi, A., Alavi, S.-S., Shakiba, A., & Salmanian, M. (2021). Prevalence of ADHD and Its Comorbidities in a Population-Based Sample. Journal of Attention Disorders, 25(8), 1058–1067. https://doi.org/10.1177/1087054719886372

Moore, L. D., Le, T., & Fan, G. (2013). DNA Methylation and Its Basic Function. Neuropsychopharmacology, 38(1), 23–38. https://doi.org/10.1038/npp.2012.112

Park, S., Lee, J.-M., Kim, J.-W., Cho, D.-Y., Yun, H. J., Han, D. H., Cheong, J. H., & Kim, B.-N. (2015). Associations between serotonin transporter gene (SLC6A4) methylation and clinical characteristics and cortical thickness in children with ADHD. Psychological Medicine, 45(14), 3009–3017. https://doi.org/10.1017/S003329171500094X

Subcommittee on Attention-Deficit/Hyperactivity Disorder, Steering Committee on Quality Improvement and Management. (2011). ADHD: Clinical Practice Guideline for the Diagnosis, Evaluation, and Treatment of Attention-Deficit/ Hyperactivity Disorder in Children and Adolescents. Pediatrics, 128(5), 1007–1022. https://doi.org/10.1542/peds.2011-2654

Takeda, T., Stotesbery, K., Power, T., Ambrosini, P. J., Berrettini, W., Hakonarson, H., & Elia, J. (2010). Parental ADHD Status and its Association with Proband ADHD Subtype and Severity. The Journal of Pediatrics, 157(6), 995-1000.e1. https://doi.org/10.1016/j.jpeds.2010.05.053

Ystrom, E., Gustavson, K., Brandlistuen, R. E., Knudsen, G. P., Magnus, P., Susser, E., Davey Smith, G., Stoltenberg, C., Surén, P., Håberg, S. E., Hornig, M., Lipkin, W. I., Nordeng, H., & Reichborn-Kjennerud, T. (2017). Prenatal Exposure to Acetaminophen and Risk of ADHD. Pediatrics, 140(5), e20163840. https://doi.org/10.1542/peds.2016-3840

Chapter 4: A discussion of Autism and its current diagnostic & treatment methods through the lens of multiculturalism

Minji Kang, HBSc (c)

Defining Autism

Autism, also often referred to as Autism Spectrum Disorder (ASD), is a developmental disability characterized in the DSM through symptoms such as: deficits in social communication, restricted/repetitive behaviors, and excessive adherence to routines. Autism Spectrum Disorder is a diagnosis which covers a spectrum of 4 more specific diagnoses, previously used by the American Psychiatric Association (APA, 2013): It covers autistic disorder, childhood disintegrative disorder, pervasive developmental disorder, and asperger's syndrome.

ASD is a disorder that is quite commonly found: 1 in 44 children in the United States are affected by this diagnosis (Autism Speaks, n.d.). Though diagnosis is most frequently made during childhood, many individuals are diagnosed later in life, and more than 5 million adults with Autism live in the US today. ASD is a disorder that affects individuals for the duration of their lives, and this makes diagnosis, intervention and education massively important for the quality of life that autistic individuals lead.

Multicultural Perceptions of Diagnosis, and Treatment

Although autism is a heavily studied and well-documented disorder, it, like many other neurodevelopmental disorders, are often lacking in its considerations for the increasingly globalizing and multicultural world we live in. Even with this understanding, three questions still remain: (1) why is there a particular emphasis on culture? (2) Why is culture something that needs to be taken into account when we are discussing neurodevelopmental disorders like ASD? (3) How can culture possibly affect things such as diagnosis, treatment and perceptions of the disorder itself?

An individual's culture is a large, inescapable part of human life. It dictates everything from social norms, core beliefs, customs, values, and many other aspects of daily life that people may not even be consciously aware of. It builds the foundations of how society perceives, and acts within the social environments. With this being said, culture is not a universal standard of operation; different regions of the world and their respective populations have varying cultural norms and practices. This variation in cultures often leads to between-culture differences in the way different neurodevelopmental disorders/invisible disabilities are perceived, addressed and managed.

These cultural differences are especially important to address for ASD for a number of reasons. First, ASD has a very complicated history of classification outside of the culturally Western diagnostic system. For many cultures, the official clinical diagnosis of ASD is a relatively new occurrence. In China, for example; ASD was not considered an official diagnosis in China until about 40 years ago (Osipsov, 2018). This recent addition of ASD as a diagnostic disorder observed in many nonwestern cultures subsequently impacts individuals in ethnic minority groups regardless of geographic location. This can be observed in the North American population- as research indicates that autism is a disorder that affects all demographic groups equally (Osipsov, 2018). However, data collected from the CDC shows that white children are more likely to be diagnosed with ASD as compared to those who are black or hispanic (CDC, 2019).

This is a potentially alarming issue, especially as additional research indicates that racial minority groups in the US are less likely to seek clinical help for the raising of autistic children, even with diagnosis (Sue & Sue, 2008). For many cultures, neurodevelopmental disorders such as ASD carry a heavy stigma- community sentiment that tends to be negative. The negative stigma varies between cultures; but it is undeniable that this negative outlook causes hesitation in the discussion or early intervention for treatment and diagnosis. This lesser likelihood to be diagnosed, along with the fact that clinical help is sought after less often, can lead to negative outcomes as early intervention is key for minimizing symptoms.

Not only are the belief systems in a culture a factor that affects the efficacy of existing diagnostic and treatment frameworks for ASD, but so are cultural differences and its impact on the presentation of symptoms in individuals from different cultures. In fact, the CDC actually suggests that cross-cultural differences may be a factor contributing to the possible underdiagnosis of ASD in ethnic minority groups in the US (CDC, 2019). The diagnostic criterion for ASD used in North America, that is, the DSM-5, mainly highlights ASD symptoms and their manifestations observed in a largely white, middle-class sample. As helpful as these diagnostic criteria may be, the somewhat rigid set of defining characteristics can sometimes act as a boundary instead of a guideline in terms of its considerations of what individuals with ASD and their caregivers may experience. This raises a number of issues especially in the wake of the rise of multiculturalism; The lack of diversity in the considerations for the presentation of symptoms in the diagnostic criterion can lead to the underdiagnosis of ASD in POC and ethnic minority groups, as symptoms may manifest differently due to the cultural norms that are enforced within specific communities.

One of the diagnostic criteria for ASD in the DSM-5: deficits in behavior used in social interaction. One of the key symptoms for this criteria is the lack of engagement in eye contact, or the impairment of the use of social eye contact. This, in the context of western cultural norms is something that may indicate deficits in social communication. However, in many East Asian cultures, avoiding eye contact with elders is an expected norm in children- these discrepancies in understood social norms therefore can result in misleading or incorrect diagnoses in these cross-cultural contexts, either from misinterpretations on the part of the professional, or on account of the parents or caregivers' lack of concern over certain symptoms due to different cultural norms (Zhang, Wheeler & Richey, 2006).

Another example is the diagnostic criterion for restrictive and repetitive behaviors (RRBIs) listed in the DSM-5. Black children were less likely than white children to have documented RRBIs in a cohort of children diagnosed with ASD, showing the inconsistency in clinical observations between the two groups (Stoll, Bergamo & Rossetti, 2021).

The disparities in access to a diagnosis and treatment don't end here. Studies show that ethnic differences can lead to referral and diagnostic biases in clinicians, with paediatricians being more likely to diagnose clinical vignettes of European babies with ASD, as compared to non-European minority cases (Begeer et al., 2009). Further, negative differences exist even within those who have been diagnosed. Research indicates that in the US, black children were on average given an ASD diagnosis later than white children, with black children having spent more time on average in treatment before a diagnosis (Mandell et al., 2002). They were also 2.6x less likely to receive a diagnosis during their first visit as compared to caucasian children (Mandell et al., 2002). This disparity in early detection and treatment of ASD only amplifies existing problems.

Another quite pronounced problem that can be encountered is the effects of language. Children and families who have immigrated from different linguistic and cultural backgrounds may have difficulties getting the help that they need, whether that be from an inability to communicate with caregivers and practitioners, or from the social and psychological pressure that may result from trying to adapt to a new cultural environment. Many individuals who operate with English as their second language may have difficulties making appointments, understanding the recommendations of treatment or voicing their needs even when care is provided (Barrio et al., 2018). Along with this, interventions for helping individuals with ASD, such as speech and language therapy, can be a source of disruption or even a loss of the first language that the child and the family of an immigrant family speaks as these interventions are almost exclusively offered in English. This can cause a plethora of problems in not only communication, but also an erasure of the sense of identity and culture that the children may have been developing (Barrio et al., 2018).

Creating a Culturally Inclusive Framework

There is an evident lack of consideration in understanding cultural values in addressing neurodevelopmental disorders such as ASD. Knowing that these knowledge gaps exist, a main priority for healthcare providers, educators, and social workers should be to have an understanding of how to build a culturally inclusive framework when meeting with ASD clients.

First and foremost, reducing stigma within different cultural communities through education and the fostering of conversations about ASD is a crucial first step. As previously discussed above, different cultures may have different levels of understanding and negative stigmas which can affect individuals' and families' willingness to seek assistance or receive a diagnosis. These stigmas can rise from a number of different sources- For example, in certain African cultures, children with ASD are seen as possessed or cursed by spirits, or as individuals affected by witchcraft (Owusu, 2021). In some Christian-dominated cultures, ASD can be seen as God's will, or even as a punishment of sorts (Barrio et al., 2018). These negative stigmas surrounding ASD causes hesitancy and shame, reducing the likelihood that individuals from these cultures will reach out for professional help, or even a diagnosis. Identifying possible barriers towards seeking clinical help within these communities such as these and addressing these barriers to create a more open and supportive attitude is necessary for a more inclusive and accessible approach. Research suggests that fostering an open conversation about child development and education (Kang-Yi et al., 2018), along with increased awareness and education about ASD as a whole, can foster positive interactions with individuals with ASD and therefore reduce stigma in these communities (Kang-Yi et al., 2018). This allows more individuals in need of diagnosis and assistance access to the care that they need.

With this, a more personal level of community also needs to be further addressed- the family or caregivers to the individuals with ASD. Many parents to children with ASD have feelings of shame, guilt or even a sense of responsibility for their children's diagnosis. Although these feelings are readily observed throughout many, if not most, parents and caregivers at one point or another, these feelings are important to address and discuss as they can have a direct impact on the children. Negative feelings, specifically shame or guilt, can cause parents and caregivers to avoid or refuse external help from other families of children with ASD- and this phenomenon is often seen in increased proportions in populations with an east asian cultural background (Barrio et al., 2018). Ethnographic research addressing personal and familial experiences regarding ASD and access to such personal accounts for parents and caregivers has also been shown to significantly help navigate what often is a stressful and foreign experience and potentially alleviate feelings of guilt or helplessness (Leonard, 1986).

It is important to note here that not all behaviors that stem from these feelings or cultural beliefs are negative. Some cultures interpret an ASD diagnosis as a blessing (Barrio et al., 2018), and different cultural beliefs and mindsets can lead to a number of different coping strategies that can benefit both the child with ASD and the rest of the family (Barrio et al., 2018), helping them lead a happier, less stressful life. However, these positive benefits of different cultural outlooks should not deter providers from ensuring that appropriate resources and knowledge is accessible to everyone.

Access to knowledge about and reducing the stigmatization around ASD for the general public is important in addition to cultural competency training for healthcare providers in the clinical setting. Research indicates that integrating a more multicultural framework for various mental disorder interventions have shown positive benefits in the past (Griner & Smith, 2006). Culturally sensitive, bottom-up approaches to treatments of major depressive disorder have shown to produce significantly better results in Latin and African American samples in the US (Kalibatseva & Leong, 2014), and many professional organizations have been adopting an increasingly culturally competent framework as an ethical obligation in the treatment of patients (Ridley, Mendoza & Kanitz, 1994).

For ASD specifically, research illatrates the use of standardized questionnaires rather than a reliance on spontaneous clinical judgements significantly decrease the disparity between ASD diagnosis for European and non-European ethnic minority groups (Begeer et al., 2009). It may be advisable, then, to introduce a simple screening list to the standard pediatric practice in order to ensure that as much clinical bias is removed from initial assessments as possible. Along with this, educating healthcare professionals who specialize in ASD in common cultural disparities in symptom manifestation, as well as how culture may influence factors such as the amount of information disclosed, ability to communicate, lack of expressions of concern over specific behaviors that may be the cultural norm, or the degree of open discussion with the medical professionals that families and individuals may provide can greatly improve the efficacy of evaluations. Overall cultural safety needs to be established in the clinical setting to improve the health outcomes for patients with ASD and other comorbidities.

ASD is a disorder that impacts a large number of people, regardless of race, gender, or cultural orientation. This makes it crucial, then, that efforts be continued in ensuring that treatment and diagnosis of ASD is more accessible, affordable and equitable for all. With a rapidly globalizing world, discussions of interculturalism, and cultural saftey are becoming more popular within the western paradigm dominated fields such as: psychology, psychiatry and all related fields is becoming more relevant than ever- and especially for disorders like ASD, where early diagnosis, treatment and intervention is crucial for a higher quality of life, it is a topic that must be addressed with urgency. Overall, improving cultural competency within all levels of providers that interact with ASD patients will work to reduce stigma, and improve health outcomes.

References

Autism statistics and facts. *Autism Speaks*. (n.d.). Retrieved July 16, 2022, from https://www.autismspeaks.org/autism-statistics-asd

Barrio, B. L., Hsiao, Y.-J., Prishker, N., & Terry, C. (2018). The impact of culture on parental perceptions about autism spectrum disorders: Striving for culturally competent practices. *Multicultural Learning and Teaching*, 14(1). https://doi.org/10.1515/mlt-2016-0010

Begeer, S., Bouk, S. E., Boussaid, W., Terwogt, M. M., Koot, H. M. (2009). Underdiagnosis and referral bias of autism in ethnic minorities. *Journal of Autism and Developmental Disorders*, 39, 142–148.

Centers for Disease Control and Prevention. (2019, August 27). *Spotlight on: Racial and ethnic differences in children identified with autism spectrum disorder (ASD).* Centers for Disease Control and Prevention. Retrieved July 20, 2022, from https://www.cdc.gov/ncbddd/autism/addm-community-report/differences-in-children.html

Griner, D., & Smith, T. B. (2006). Culturally adapted mental health intervention: A meta-analytic review. *Psychotherapy: Theory, Research, Practice, Training*, 43(4), 531–548. \ https://doi.org/10.1037/0033-3204.43.4.531

Kalibatseva, Z., & Leong, F. T. (2014). A critical review of culturally sensitive treatments for depression: Recommendations for intervention and research. *Psychological Services, 11*(4), 433–450. https://doi.org/10.1037/a0036047

Kang-Yi, C. D., Grinker, R. R., Beidas, R., Agha, A., Russell, R., Shah, S. B., Shea, K., & Mandell, D. S. (2018). Influence of community-level cultural beliefs about autism on families' and professionals' care for children. *Transcultural Psychiatry*, 55(5), 623–647. https://doi.org/10.1177/1363461518779831

Leonard, J. H. (1986). Families and autism: An ethnographic approach. Dissertation Abstracts International, 47, 2333

Mandell, D. S., Listerud, J., Levy, S. E., & Pinto-Martin, J. A. (2002). Race differences in the age at diagnosis among medicaid-eligible children with autism. *Journal of the American Academy of Child and Adolescent Psychiatry*, 41(12), 1447–1453. https://doi-org.myaccess.library.utoronto.ca/10.1097/00004583-200212000-00016

Osipsov, D. (2018). Multicultural Perspectives on Autism Spectrum Disorder. *The Complexity of Autism Spectrum Disorders*, 148–155. https://doi.org/10.4324/9780429454646-9

Owusu, B. A. (2021). Perceived causes and diagnosis of febrile convulsion in selected rural contexts in Cape Coast Metropolis, Ghana. https://doi.org/10.21203/rs.3.rs-929178/v1

Ridley C, Mendoza D, Kanitz B. Multicultural training: reexamination, operationalization, and integration. *Couns. Psychol.* 1994;22:227–289

Stoll, M. M., Bergamo, N., & Rossetti, K. G. (2021). Analyzing modes of assessment for children with autism spectrum disorder (ASD) using a culturally sensitive lens. Advances in Neurodevelopmental Disorders, 5(3), 233–244. https://doi.org/10.1007/s41252-021-00210-0

Sue, D. W., Sue, D. (2008). Counseling the culturally diverse: Theory and practice (5th ed.). Hoboken, NJ: John Wiley.

Zhang, J., Wheeler, J. J., & Richey, D. (2006). Cultural validity in assessment instruments for children with autism from a Chinese cultural perspective. *International Journal of Special Education*, 21(1), 109–114

Chapter 5: A Personal Reflection on Being a Young Neurodiverse Professional Navigating Higher Education and Labor Force

Lydia C. Rehman HBSc., MPH (c)

Neurodiversity in Post-Secondary Education

Being a neurodiverse person comes with its many strengths, but various social factors can make it exhausting to manage what should be daily life. For instance, workplaces, education systems, and society are not naturally designed to accommodate and support neurodivergent people or people with mental health disabilities. For context, I am a graduate student living with ADHD and attending a leading global institution, how I got to this stage is remarkable, and the only memory I have of getting to this level of what you may call "success" is through struggle. Many of my struggles with ADHD have been masked by an invisible mental health disability and both were diagnosed recently. In this paper I will outline my experience(s) of being neurodiverse as a student in post-secondary education, and being a young professional in the labor force.

While the impacts of having multiple invisible disabilities have impacted the entirety of my life, the recognizability of it did not begin until orientation week of my first year of university. It wasn't until this week that I self-recognized triggers: for example, loud music, over-stimulation, and forced participation; at times, aggravated me without an understanding of why. However, despite all these feelings,

I felt an immense pressure to act "normal" and because I had all these different needs or struggles, I ended up not participating in many of the further events, or if I tried to attend some social events it would be overstimulating and I would be required to leave.

This experience set the trajectory for the next three years within the higher education system. I was a "pre-med" student, and my classes were challenging for numerous reasons. My energy levels constantly fluctuate; given that my energy can become very low fast, my motivation becomes limited. It's difficult to function when you don't have energy or motivation, for even the most basic tasks. It's exhausting to wake up and not be able to do the basic activities such as brushing your teeth, eating, let alone starting a project, and it's a constant cycle that ends in self-loathing and embarrassment when you have to take responsibility for lost time. Further, sitting in a class was at-times unbearable; having to sit in a classroom with constant distractions and ways of becoming overstimulated is something not easy to manage. The lecture halls are overwhelmingly massive. I have various sensory issues that can overwhelm me, and within the classroom it was hard to not become overwhelmed. For example, people would often be sat close together, I could hear chewing, pencil tapping, the lecture itself. The lights and the alarming number of noises trigger my sensory issues to the point where I can't take notes, function, or even think. It becomes a matter of needing to get out of the situation and environment. This isn't great because many courses take attendance, and students are required to be there, and some professors can be very vocal about students who leave classes halfway through or don't show up; sometimes, it can be tremendously stress-inducing.

Part of my mental health disability includes anxiety, and having anxiety and ADHD is an interesting soup combination. On the one hand, you love academia, and learning, but having ADHD and multiple assignments to complete makes it unbearable at times to start your tasks, and follow through without any motivation. Likewise, your crippling anxiety becomes stressed if it doesn't get done and submitted on time: So, on the day before something is due, you wait until midnight to begin your assignment and hyperfocus until it's done. I have learned to understand that I am more than just being "lazy", I recently learned from a healthcare provider that the reason I will purposely stress myself out to complete a task, is because stress releases dopamine, and dopamine is what I need to focus and get tasks done.

Hyperfocus is an interesting thing, and it's a superpower, as it gives you the capacity to have an intense concentration for many hours (Nadeau, 2016). Imagine being able to get done a 10-page well-researched academic paper in 3 hours. As efficient as it may sound, it's exhausting; I tend to hyperfocus on things I don't need to do. For example, if something excites me such as applying to a new job, joining a student club, becoming a committee member, than it's exciting for me to sit and apply until it's done.

At the beginning of university in 2016, I never heard much from professors or staff about accessibility services, nor was I encouraged to take care of my mental health within the academic institution. What I did hear though, is that "only a number of you are going to survive this class." There's nothing like being made to feel like another number in a system of competition. Professors made these classes seem so "cutthroat," and that they were. I wish there had been better advocacy and encouragement to seek help through academic accomadations, to receive assistance with learning difficulties as a result of neurodevelopmental and mental health disorders. Perhaps then, I could've been better equipped to handle the pretentious reputation of the western academic institution.

On this idea of handling the nature of an academic environment, many students are competitive in everything they do. Everyone is on the road to medical, law, graduate school and getting there means to get the best internships and volunteer positions. Here's a word of advice for others who feel overwhelmed by the pressure of academia, worry less. Everyone has their path, even if it is like a poorly constructed road. Most people do not finish a degree in "4 years" which is completely respectable. I didn't get as far as I did because I had a 4.0 grade point average. I just pushed myself to get involved with campus life, and step outside of an extremely comfortable bubble. This self-encouragement pushed me to want to do better, to not let my social anxiety and fear of rejection consume me from having the best possible university experience. I foraged new relationships with professors, which brought new opportunities. In 2020 when COVID-19 pandemic began, it really changed my life. I became president of an academic student society. I thrived in the virtual environment because I could do my work at my own pace, in my own space, in what made me feel most comfortable. I never realized how much more I could accomplish, and I ended up getting into a graduate program at a top institution.

Multi-potentiality is an interesting concept, in short, it means that you are a person that isn't destined for one position, one career, and one life focus. You are an individual who may be well-rounded and highly skilled, not just in one area, but it also means that you may need to constantly change your current priorities and focus (WTY, 2018). What is interesting is when you are an individual who has multi-potentiality, and ADHD associated decision paralysis, meaning that it's extremely difficult, if not impossible, to decide upon a decision due to how your brain thinks. I am privileged to have developed years of skills, and education in all different areas. Everything excites me, and can be really stimulating, thus I tend to crave to learn more without taking any breaks.

When I get asked the question: " So what's next after you get your undergraduate degree?" I say, "I don't know." They ask again. "What next after your masters." Now I've concluded that when I am asked, I tell people: "I want to be a barbie with 500+ careers." People who may be neurotypical may not understand, but it's difficult to choose one life trajectory when you need constant excitement to have the motivation to move forward with one thing. By one thing, I mean career, job, and hobbies. I didn't get diagnosed with ADHD until later in life, and there are many things now I look back on and reflect upon how I didn't recognize the signs earlier in life.

Neurodiversity in the Workplace

As previously outlined, being neurodiverse in the education system is challenging, however it's a similar experience in the workplace, especially when workplaces may not be equipped to meet your individual needs. Neurodiversity is a term that collectively describes people who think differently (Burnett, 2019). I have been privileged to work from home since the start of the COVID-19 pandemic. Teleworking has been a major strength for my ADHD as I can create my own workspace that is comfortable and in essence work with complete flexibility. I tend to get bursts of energy at nighttime, so from 9 pm - 3am may be my most productive hours of the day, or at least hours where I am most inclined to be productive. While COVID-19 has been a debilitating nightmare, I never knew how much I needed this flexibility in my life. This flexibility provides me with a capacity to strive on my own terms, however despite having the flexibility sometimes starting even the most basic of tasks can be of great difficulty; and working from home as a neurodivergent person just means that there may be about ten times more distractions and a consistent lack of motivation to do work.

Many adults with ADHD struggle with fluctuating energy levels, when there is a need to engage in mental activity that requires full concentration (Nadeau, 2016). This is my own experience, and based upon the literature, simple changes that can be implemented in the workplace include flexibility in working hours, and a need for employers understand that individuals who are neurodivergent may have days where the employee may be perfectly able to complete their job, but not always within the physical working environment. Employers should try to be more creative with the physical workspace by implementing spaces that may be either more quiet or creative in nature (Burnett, 2019). Further, being clear and direct can be helpful, as not everyone is able to work without clear direction (Burnett, 2019). Based upon my own experience, employers often don't understand how making the workplace (eg. physical space, communication, activities) inclusive can actually allow someone with neurodivergence to thrive and exceed company/self productivity (Burnett, 2019)

As previously mentioned, through my previous education, research and work experience I have developed a strong set of skills that make me a well-rounded indvidual. Thus, finding one life focus is of too much difficulty, becoming bored in jobs can happen fairly quickly. This is because when applying to a position, or any opportunity I am excited about starting, but can get bored very easily because my brain seeks instant gratification, and when that is not recieved my ADHD brain is inclined to look for the next exciting opportunity to repeat this endless debilitating cycle. This is what is referred to as "Impulsive Job Hopping" which is where an individual may say yes to an opportunity before waiting to analyze a job's suitability (Nadeau, 2016). Further, in doing so you promise a lot more than you may be able to deliver (Nadeau, 2016). This can be a really difficult process, consequently, there's immense shame associated with having to explain to your supervisor why you were unable to fulfill the tasks that you promised you could do with confidence. However I try hard to fuel the boredom that I may feel, I turn what may be seen as a deficit or negative attitude to channel creative ideas in order to innovate the work being done. My brain acts as a catalyst for an idea generator, and as a young person in the labor force, my ideas have not always been valued, which is extremely discouraging to continue work in that particular space, especially when your ideas are highly innovative and aim to transform your work.

Overall, the workplace isn't always understanding of what your disability is, what it entails, thus there are typically limited policies that work to accommodate invisible disabilities. Most workplaces tailor the environment to what is most convenient to the majority rather than individualize the work environment (Burnett, 2019). It also is a completely nerve-racking experience to disclose a disability, because subconsciously social norms have rooted my thinking that outing my disability would be a burden to the productivity of a corporation. Further, I am constantly worried that me sharing my disability, or requiring accommodations would result in a termination. However, understanding life experiences, and research looking at the strengths of ADHD has made me realize how important neurodivergence is within the workplace. I have a very creative mind, and I can think in special ways that look at ideas from a different perspective, I aim extremely high, and with the right workplace, my ambition can strive.

References

Burnett, K. (2019). Embracing Neurodiversity in the workplace. *Training Journal*, http://myaccess.library.utoronto.calogin?qurl=https%3A%2F%2Fwww.proquest.com%2Ftrade-journals%2Fembracing-neurodiversity-workplace%2Fdocview%2F2304074885%2Fse-2

Nadeau, K. G. (2016). The ADHD guide to career success : harness your strengths, manage your challenges (2nd ed.). Routledge. https://doi.org/10.4324/9781315723334

(WTY). "Are You A Multipotentialite? A TED Talk On Why Some of Us Don't Have One True Calling." *Watch The Yard*, 5 July 2018, www.watchtheyard.com/education/multipotentialite-polymath

Chapter 6: A Personal Reflection on being Neurodiverse: Challenges, Treatment, Co-morbidities and Barriers within Higher Education as a Mature Post-Secondary Student

Mustafa Abbas Zain, HBA (c)

Neurodiversity, Comorbidities and the Deficit Driven Diagnostic Criteria

Neurodivergence is an incredibly vast and diverse subject; it's more of an umbrella term that covers multiple experiences that are subdivided by specific diagnostic classifications. Perhaps this holistic approach actively challenges conventional thought on the origins of neuro-developmental "disorders" and their overlapping characteristics. The idea centrally revolves around the mutual co-existence of different symptoms in varying degrees (Clouder et al., 2020). While the concept of neurodiversity has been widely discussed in detail in earlier chapters of this book, it is important to mention how these ideas materialized and surfaced. In this chapter, I will reflect on my experiences as a neurodivergent individual who is incidentally an immigrant and a mature student, including navigating diagnosis, treatment, and barriers within a well-renowned post-secondary institution.

As a person with lived experience with neurodivergence, looking at it from a medical or diagnostic standpoint can seriously overlook

A Personal Reflection on being Neurodiverse: Challenges, Treatment... 59

how it affects a person. The word "divergence" means difference and cannot be reduced to a universal set of symptoms. To further this, the concept of neurodiversity focuses on accepting greater intersectionality within various disorders such as ADHD, Autistic Spectrum Disorder , Asperger's Syndrome, and Tourette's Syndrome. The idea behind the diagnostic modalities relies on only treating symptoms. More specifically, Dr. Gabor Mate provides a discussion on ADHD/ADD to discuss beyond the genetic and biological factors of the disorder itself. Instead, he focuses on socio-economic factors, which later get molded as a behavioral response to life situations that stem from early childhood development and environmental factors (Mate, 2021). Further, Dr. Mate details each individual's innate bio-physiological predispositions, which are shaped by a child's ability to respond to certain stimuli on a threshold that may be higher or lower compared to other neurotypical peers (Mate, 2021). He also notes that early childhood trauma heavily influences the ability to respond and develop habits that could alleviate the impacts.

Understanding Co-morbidities, and Reflecting on Social Identity and Navigating Diagnosis, Treatment

Understanding the neurodivergent experience can be difficult as there are a multitude of accessibility barriers, in addition to having 'comorbidities' or multple coexisting conditions. It is first important to define co-morbidities in the context of neurodivergence. In addition to having one disease/disorder, such as ADHD, many individuals may also have multiple coexisting diseases (Valderas et al., 2009). One of the issues with having several concurrent diseases/conditions/disorders simultaneously is that there is limited research and understanding of how people with comorbidities view their illnesses. However, understanding the morbidity burden is essential, which assesses the impact and severity for the person with multiple existing conditions (Valderas et al., 2009). These burdens are influenced by socioeconomic, cultural, and environmental factors (Valderas et al., 2009). In terms of my journey with neurodivergence and other coexisting conditions, one factor I have noticed is the lack of cultural relevance/competency by healthcare and education professionals. Further, I have experienced a consistent lack of understanding of the severity of the different conditions, and medical providers lack the patient experience, and the cultural values of the patient themselves.

Journeying into Post-Secondary Education

My first attempt at seeking a diagnosis for my learning challenges began with a conversation with the administrative staff at the Toronto Adult Learning Center (ALC); this experience was rooted in the dismissal and gaslighting of my experiences. The adult learning center was situated in a low-income, refugee-populated area. Having my concerns invalidated was a shock, as I expected staff to have better empathy and understanding of immigrants and BIPOC health. While this experience was disheartening as a recent immigrant, and to have traumatic experiences within, I decided it was best to continue my courses at the adult learning center so that I could reach my goal of getting accepted into a post-secondary education.

Within a month of completing the pre-requisite course at the ALC, I was admitted to one of the leading universities in Canada, where I felt genuinely welcomed and grateful that my prior education, and life experiences were considered to provide me with an offer-of-admission. I was overly ambitious and thought I was secure in understanding my academic interests and future goals. I decided upon courses and enrolled myself part-time, which would allow me greater flexibility with my accessibility needs for being neurodivergent and an immigrant with various cultural and family responsibilities.

As I was progressing through my first semester, I began noticing challenges that impacted my ability to provide quality sufficient academic output. I was overstaying lengthy hours at the library following classes, reading course material on the bus, and re-reading assignments on my way to work. My grades remained low, and grasping material was very challenging. I tried different techniques and began engaging with my professors and course teaching assistants (TAs); I went to office hours and extra writing sessions run by an academic writing center. It was exhausting to know the effort I was putting in compared to the reality of my grades and ability to complete work. Nevertheless, I chose not to give up because I had to come very far in my life to get the opportunity to study at this top institution. It wasn't until one of the course TAs shared their similar experience of being a BIPOC student with multiple neurodevelopmental disabilities that they recommended I reach out to the school's department of accessibility.

While trying to deal with the burden of enrolling in accessibility services, I managed work, family, and school to the best of my ability, but things became more overwhelming. I was consistently late to classes, began making careless mistakes within my assignments, and managing time and appointments was extremely difficult. I lived a disordered life that went undiagnosed for so long that it was difficult for me to recognize that it wasn't just a matter of me "not trying hard enough".

Upon finally making the appointment with accessibility services to receive academic accommodations, I was provided with a stack of papers that needed to be filled by a qualified healthcare professional. These papers included a "certificate of disability", which highlights what conditions/disabilities you have that limit your academic functioning. As a newcomer to Canada, getting acquainted with life was a difficult transition. I was unaware I needed a family doctor, one who could have filled out the necessary forms. Given that I didn't have a family doctor, I decided to walk to a nearby walk-in clinic to fill out the accessibility forms. Given that I didn't have a family doctor, I decided to walk to a nearby walk-in clinic to fill out the accessibility forms. Unfortunately, the physician refused to fill the forms and claimed it would be too much of a liability. This process was tremendously frustrating that I decided to give up on the academic accommodations for the rest of the year as the tasks associated were not without barriers. My academic and learning struggle only worsened after my choice not to move forward with filling out the necessary paperwork to get accommodations. A major barrier to getting diagnosed with neurodevelopmental disorders as an adult is that it's extremely expensive.

I decided that I could not continue my post-secondary education without assistance from the university accessibility services, as my diagnosis with ADHD and other comorbidities were having a significant impact on my academic abilities. The academic advisor that I was assigned to was one of the most understanding people I had communicated with throughout my educational journey. The advisor was empathic and supportive of me processing the initial diagnosis. Further as I previously mentioned, getting tested for neurodevelopmental disorders as an adult is costly, and she ensured that I was able to attain funding for me to complete psychoeducation assessments to diagnose my neurodevelopmental disorders.

Academic Accommodations, and Systemic Barriers in Post-Secondary Education

Initially the academic accommodations were helpful in supporting my academic needs as a result of my many co-existing conditions. As a social sciences and humanities student going through the higher education system, managing treatment, having full-time employment, and managing academics, is tremendously difficult. Moreover, my experience with the onset of the COVID-19 pandemic and the transition to virtual learning, and support was highly inaccessible. It should be noted that the current educational system in a broader context is not well designed to support the needs of mature students, nor mature students with various disabilities. As a neurodivergent student in an inaccessible system is incredibly debilitating and hinders my growth as an aspiring professional.

Completing accommodation requests is a laborious administrative process. You have to prepare the list of all courses with their specific deadlines, which includes formulating specific course guidelines, following up, and writing down each particular test date and assignment date where you may be able to request accommodation/follow up with professors. These tasks multiply when you're a student with accessibility needs; this is an additional burden on the actual learning process as it requires time to learn the material, complete the corresponding assignments, and seek office hours to seek clarity on course assignments from professors. Naturally, this often becomes an overwhelming process where multiple timelines are close by with equal importance. The trauma response of flight or freeze can activate, depriving one of valuable time and resources.Symptoms such as time blindness, task paralysis, and added anxiety all drain the neurodivergent mind. All this energy, if saved, could be allocated to other parts of academic learning. The responsibility of action, timelines, and accuracy are burdened upon the same student requesting support in the same things they may not be able to do similarly as their neurotypical peers who may have been much more comfortable being able to work through such processes. While support is present but, I find the model obsolete. The technological barriers can often become a timesink where you have to spend countless hours configuring minute details like learning to navigate the library website and successfully cite academic references.

Based upon my own experience with the accessibility services at the university, its evident that their working model is best for supporting students who have been diagnosed earlier in life, and those that have more extensive social supports Neurodivergence is something that should be embraced for the strengths it holds, but also recognize the barriers to everyday life. Finding support to navigate through the education systems have continuously exposed me to various barriers that have impeded on my abilities to thrive.

Receiving a diagnosis later in life is frustrating as you have to address many of the struggles, strengths, and ultimately learning to manage on your own for the first time. Whereas, my peers with an early diagnosis had access to individualized attention from the elementary school level; having an Individualized Educational Plan (IEP), as narrated, helped them navigate academic overwhelm with more support. An early diagnosis with a neurodevelopmental disorder would mean that they would have had higher exposure to coaching, therapy, and other supports to assist in guiding their life choices in their trajectories to post-secondary education.

The current accessibility system continues to rely on archaic infrastructure (eg. reductionist treatment models) than genuine acceptance, inclusion, and equity is less likely to be attained. Regardless of age of diagnosis, many of my peers who are neurodivergent note similar struggles. This itself is indicative that innovative and inclusive solutions need to continually be developed to meet the diverse needs of students with neurodivergence. One issue that many only understand is ADHD as a neurological disorder, and they only highlight the symptoms of ADHD. Developing a refined view of ADHD requires education systems to put more effort into understanding how individual ADHD manifests and how individual capacity and responsibility to manage the disorder are highly diverse in individuals. (Nadeau, 2016).

Based upon my experience in higher education has allowed me to realize that I should not have to mask who I am as a neurodivergent person, immigrant, and mature student to fit the norms of society. The act of masking itself is a trauma response which neurodivergent people have to indulge to blend in. The act of masking can be defined as behaving in ways that appear normal as a means of socializing and being accepted within society. Seeking accommodations are on a need-to know basis as there are certain risks involved with seeking support. Once things are documented, due to the level of stigma that exists in society, there can be repercussions or discrimination within the workplace or education system for people who are neurodivergent or have invisible disabilities. Society needs to work towards becoming a society that is both trauma and culturally informed.

It can be almost traumatizing to individuals with neurodivergence or invisible disabilities when language is non-inclusive, nor trauma/culture-informed. For example, the simple way we phrase 'impairment' in relation to neurodivergence can be harmful, as it shouldn't only be addressed from this lens; it should recognize its variability in each individual. As stigma exists, and being able to provide authentic inclusion based on compassion and understanding is what is necessary for supporting the diverse needs of individuals. Lastly, those with neurodivergence have incredible strengths that are of tremendous value in education systems, labor-force and the broader context of society.

References

Clouder, Karakus, M., Cinotti, A., Ferreyra, M. V., Fierros, G. A., & Rojo, P. (2020). Neurodiversity in higher education: a narrative synthesis. *Higher Education, 80(4),* 757–778. https://doi.org/10.1007/s10734-020-00513-6

Mate. G (2021, August 18). AD(H)D. Retrieved from https://drgabormate.com/adhd/

Valderas, J. M., Starfield, B., Sibbald, B., Salisbury, C., & Roland, M. (2009). Defining Comorbidity: Implications for Understanding Health and Health Services. Annals of Family Medicine, 7(4), 357–363. https://doi.org/10.1370/afm.983

Nadeau, K. G. (2016). The ADHD guide to career success : harness your strengths, manage your challenges (2nd ed.). Routledge.doi.org/10.4324/9781315723334

Chapter 7: Health Promotion and Stigma in Neurodiversity

Natanel Krieksfeld

Defining Stigma

When people fall outside of the standard social norms, they are often characterized as being different (Nerenberg, 2021). Stigma is where an individual may view another person in a particular way that is negative, due to having some personal characteristics that may be seen as either a :disadvantage or stereotype (Mayo Clinic, 2017). Stigma can be extremely harmful to individuals who are neurodiverse or have invisible disabilities as it may result in hesitancy to seek care. Further it may result in bullying, violence or low-self confidence due to the lack of understanding from people within a social environment (Mayo Clinic, 2017).

Common Myths & Stereotypes about Neurodivergence & Mental Illness

Within disorders that are characterized as "neurodivergent" there are many common stereotypes, and myths that create stigma about particular disorders. For example in ADHD there are various common myths which include: (1) ADHD is a non-existent disorder, and that is over-diagnosed (2) ADHD disorder always begins and is diagnosed in childhood (4). Kids that have ADHD are more medicated than they need to be (5). Poor parenting is the cause for ADHD (6). Youth are overdiagnosed and overmedicated (7). Women and girls have lowered rates of ADHD compared to men and boys (POP, 2021). Despite the stigma that exists, society does not have an understanding that individuals who have ADHD may manifest certain traits uniquely, and it should not be generalized. Thus, reducing stigma requires; individuals, educators, healthcare professionals, community service workers, education systems and the workplace to become knowledgeable on neurodivergence and invisible disabilities. Reducing stigma and harmful narratives for neurodivergent disorders is essential to improving mental and physical health outcomes.

Autism & Stigma

Autism is a neurodevelopmental disorder that has different groups of characteristics. One of the main characteristics of autism include difficulties within social interactions (Donohue, 2019). One way to reduce the stigma that exists towards autism is for those who are non-autistic to improve personal social awareness. Society needs to become understanding of the diversity amongst people in the classroom, workplace and any space where autistic people are. People with autism are more likely to be predisposed to other mental health issues as a result of potential struggles of being on the spectrum. On this notion of a spectrum, society needs to be aware that not all autistic people can not be reduced to a universal set of symptoms. Autism is more than an illness, and that there should be a more strengths-based-approach when having conversations surrounding the topic (Sussex, n.d.).

ADHD & Stigma

ADHD stands for Attention Deficit Hyperactivity Disorder. ADHD is also a neurodevelopmental disorder that commonly manifests in childhood, and can impact a person throughout the duration of their life. Some common characteristics of ADHD include: an inability to maintain attention and concentration with required tasks. As outlined in previous chapters there are different types of ADHD and can also be associated with hyperactive behavior. (Smith, 2022). There are a lot of ways to reduce the stigma that exists surrounding ADHD, of which includes: educating society, and workplaces about what the needs of people with ADHD may be (POP, 2021). For those who have ADHD, finding community is important to further assist with mitigating the impacts of the disorder. There also needs to be reduction in stigma surrounding medication, as ADHD is typically a disorder that requires a combination of medication and different types of behavioral therapy. There should be further health promotion activities to ensure that people are aware that medication is used to help people, and that there is no shame in seeking help. Overall ADHD is a disorder that can severely limit an individual's capacity to flourish when there is a lack of understanding of what the disorder/disability entails from workplaces and education.

Therapy

Therapy is an important factor for individuals with neurodevelopmental, mental health and other invisible disabilities. As previously mentioned, as a consequent result people who are neurodivergent are reluctant to seek therapy due to the level of shame or stigma that exists (Mayo Clinic, 2017). Much of this shame exists because of years of societal ignorance, and a lack of willingness for people to admit their needs. As a result people who do undertake therapy may be afraid to share their stories with healthcare providers about their struggles with mental health, or other neurodivergent disorders as they fear being judged, and having their feelings dismissed. Another issue which may arise from undergoing therapeutic treatment is that it is not something that is easily accessible, nor affordable to people who need it the most (Sussex, n.d.). Furthermore, people who need to seek therapy may not have insurance that covers the expensive costs. There are limited programs that fund these opportunities especially for those who receive a diagnosis in adulthood. For individuals that live in remote or rural areas, access to services is difficult as there are limited resources and a larger demand for services. Overall without having access to therapy, health outcomes with the associated mental health, or neurodevelopmental disorders can be poor.

One factor that should be considered is reframing the idea of therapy and health, and how to, although therapy is a subjective topic, because managing a disorder works best based on what the individual's needs are. For example, within research in the field of psychotherapy there was a study conducted on goal focused positive psychotherapy (GFPP) (Conoley, 2019). This type of positive therapy explores what patients are capable of accomplishing when they are able to harness emotions, strengths and goals that are positive in nature (Conoley, 2019). This success allows for therapists to harness a strengths based approach and focus on the patients set of strengths (Conoley, 2019).

There are various types of therapy, and one of them is Cognitive Behavioral Therapy (CBT). CBT is a type of short-term treatment which helps people to be able to solve problems. CBT also helps to reveal the relationships between beliefs, thoughts, feelings, and the behaviors which may follow as a result of those relationships. Another type of therapy is Dialectical Behavioral Therapy (DBT). DBT is a modified form of CBT. DBT teaches people how to live in the current moment, how to develop efficient ways to cope with stress, as well as, regulate their emotions and improve their relationships with others. One treatment is by undertaking pharmacotherapy to manage signs and symptoms with antipsychotic medications (Serene Life Hospital team, 2012). An additional treatment is psychotherapy which helps an individual to learn how to take control of his/her/their own life and learn to respond to various challenging situations with healthy coping skills (Serene Life Hospital, 2012). Another treatment is to undertake relapse prevention training (RPT) (Serene Life Hospital, 2012). This type of training is an approach used by healthcare providers to work with patients to identify triggers of a possible relapse. It should be noted that relapse is a large part of a person's recovery process when dealing with mental illnesses, substance abuse disorders and other coexisting conditions (RPT, 2022). This training allows people to strategize ways in identifying early warning signs, and potential triggers. (RPT, 2022). This approach helps the individual to develop coping strategies, and takes a strengths-based-approach to assist with skills development and promoting healthy recovery (RPT, 2022).

Mental Health and Issues & ADHD in the Workplace

Humans naturally are inclined to work to fulfill a sense of life purpose, however as individuals enter the workforce, the demand of the labor market is in a major public health crisis as people are pressured to manage high workloads (Quelch & Knoop, 2018). It is suggested that how managers in the workplace choose to learn and become educated on mental health issues and how to create the best practices for having safe and manageable workplaces can have a huge impact for the broader organization and community (Quelch & Knoop, 2018). Having a mental illness causes impairments to an individual's cognitive functions that makes it difficult to perform within an economy that is reliant on brain power (Quelch & Knoop, 2018). It can be extremely difficult for individuals to hide their mental health disabilities due to the fact that hiding underperformance can't be done easliy. While there is heavy stigma associated with mental illness, environments are getting progressively better at addressing mental health, and building increased education, and awareness. For example: medications such as antidepressants are becoming less stigmatized and more understood (Quelch & Knoop, 2018). In addition to having a mental health disability or invisible disability, there is a strong correlation that the workplace also adds to the impacts of an existing invisible or physical disability (Quelch & Knoop, 2018). Further working can act as a catalyst to reduce individuals' well-being as job stress can further impact mental health. There is current legislation in place to ensure that employees are not discriminated against due to ability, and mental health status, however many of these policies could be expanded to offer improved accommodations and full protection against workplace discrimination (Quelch & Knoop, 2018). Based on literature, one recommendation to improve awareness about mental health in the workplace includes expanding efforts to promote mindfulness, and well-being activities/incentives for employees (Quelch & Knoop, 2018). It is also noted that workers are less likely to disclose their illnesses or disorders leading to feeling misunderstood. Further, there is a constant fear of repercussion for those with mental illnesses as managers may have a personality in the workplace that lacks emotional intelligence. Further having managers that are able to be self-reflective about their own biases is important in creating safe and healthy environments that meet the individual needs of all its employees (Quelch & Knoop, 2018).

Literature suggests that ADHD in the workplace can be very difficult for building interpersonal relations, having efficient communication, managing stress and fulfilling job duties (Nadeau, 2016). Women with ADHD are more likely to face a number of challenges compared to their male counterparts. For example they have a higher likelihood of being hired to complete jobs that require the skill of being highly detail oriented (Nadeau, 2016). Further, for women who have families, managing home life and work life can be difficult (Nadeau, 2016). Social expectations in the workplace can be different and there may be increased negative attitudes when there are traits of ADHD displayed. Workplaces should ensure that they are working from an inclusive framework so that all employees regardless of ability are protected and accommodated based on their needs (Nadeau, 2016).

Assessing Empathy & Strengths Based Approaches as Health Promotion
Overall, people that are neurodivergent are individually unique, however having empathy as a care provider is important to increase the

quality of healthcare and interactions between patients and providers (Burks & Kobus, 2012). Further one study suggests that as medical students progress in their education, and clinical training they become more prone to a culture of burnout, cynicism, and demonstrate a more negative detachment from their work. However with proper mentorship, and guidance from senior clinicians, they can develop listening skills that are reflective, as well as developing understanding for patients that are non-verbal. Overall, there needs to be greater empathy and kindness provided to individuals on all levels (Burks & Kobus, 2012). Many of these disorders can lead to low-self confidence, and having dismissive attitudes towards people due to neurodivergence can be extremely hurtful, and lead to lower life quality and poor health outcomes (Burks & Kobus, 2012). Qualitative research highlights that therapists, psychiatrists, and social workers are also in major need of education as there has been instances of providers being worried about angering a patient, or their family; in the provider being reluctant to refer a patient to a specialist to be diagnosed with a neurodevelopmental disability or mental illness. Not providing quality care due to the stigmatization of disorders can impact an individual's life, as these disorders affect throughout the duration of their life. Ensuring that the patient has the autonomy to discover, learn and adapt to their diagnosed disorder is important in reframing the concept of what makes a person healthy (Nerenberg, 2021).

Society generally lacks an understanding of what it's like to be neurodivergent, and this lack of understanding, in addition to implicit bias creates stigma, and reinforces narrative stereotypes. A tremendous amount of research is being done in the area of positive psychology which looks at how interventions within education are increasingly improving a system built on negative stereotypes and bigotry. Further this field is being applied in youth development, and within the classroom which is important because its a type of therapy that harnesses the strengths of a disorder, disease, condition, or disability, and uses those strengths to develop new relationships and pathways for clients and their therapists to live through a framework of wellness and not illness (Conoley, 2019).

Anthropologist Roy Grinker suggests that his research shows that in order to reframe discussions surrounding mental illness, neurodiversity society needs to look at the historical perceptions of mental illness (Nerenberg, 2021). Stigma towards mental illness specifically has different causes depending on the country, region and varying cultural norms (Nerenberg, 2021). For example, what society may not be consciously aware of is the fact that mental illness was seen at the early beginning of capitalism (Nerenberg, 2021). As some workers were notably unable to produce as an "autonomous" person (Nerenberg, 2021). This ideology further explains why stigma for disorders such as schizophrenia or substance use tend to be higher, because they hinder those ideas of productivity and self control that are rooted in the values of capitalism (Nerenberg, 2021). He highlights that one of the issues that further perpetuates stigma is the fact that society talks about mental illness, and disability as a foreign, scary or taboo topic (Nerenberg, 2021). Whereas these ideas are why stigma exists in the first place, the goal should be for there to be health promotion campaigns that provide education on disability, mental illness and neurodivergence need to increase (Nerenberg, 2021).

Overall, society is composed of individuals that are neurotypical, or neurodivergent, and mental illness exists within both of those categories. Reframing the way discussions are held surrounding these topics is essential to reduce stigma, and overall improve the well-being of individuals. Simple words can be the difference between sharing harmful narratives, and educating others out of ignorance. As previously mentioned, invisible disabilities are not always physical or visible, so ensuring communication with others, should be respectful and with the understanding that everyone goes through unique life experiences, and being open-minded and self-reflective is what makes a person well-rounded and necessary in creating better life quality for others.

References:

Burks, D. J., & Kobus, A. M. (2012). The legacy of altruism in health care: the promotion of empathy, prosociality and humanism. Medical Education, 46(3), 317–325. https://doi.org/10.1111/j.1365-2923.2011.04159.x

Conoley, C. W. Collie W., & Scheel, M. J. (2018). Goal focused positive psychotherapy : a strengths-based approach. Oxford University Press.

Higuera, V. (2021). Everything you want to know about depression. Healthline. Retrieved August 11, 2022, from https://www.healthline.com/health/depression https://doi.org/10.1111/j.1365-2923.2011.04159.x

Mayo Clinic (2017). Mental health: Overcoming the stigma of mental illness.. Retrieved from https://www.mayoclinic.org/diseases-conditions/mental-illness/in-depth/mental-health/art-20046477

Nadeau, K. G. (2016). The ADHD guide to career success : harness your strengths, manage your challenges (2nd ed.). Routledge. https://doi.org/10.4324/9781315723334

Nerenberg J.(n.d.). How to Dismantle the Stigma of Mental Illness. Retrieved from https://greatergood.berkeley.edu/article/item/how_to_dismantle_the_stigma_of_erapy

PowerofPositivity (POP). (2021). What is it really like to live with mental illness? Power of Positivity: Positive Thinking & Attitude. Retrieved August 11, 2022, from https://www.powerofpositivity.com/what-its-like-live-with-mental-illness/

(RPT) Relapse Prevention Training. (2022, May 19). Retrieved from https://practicetransformation.umn.edu/practice-tools/relapse-prevention-training/#:~:text=Relapse prevention training is an,different things to different people.

Smith, M. (2022). Living well with a disability. HelpGuide.org. Retrieved August 11, 2022, from https://www.helpguide.org/articles/healthy-living/living-well-with-a-disability.htm

Sussex Publishers. (n.d.). The biggest problem in therapy. Psychology Today. Retrieved August 11, 2022, from https://www.psychologytoday.com/us/blog/anxiety-zen/201606/the-biggest-problem-in-

Quelch, J. A., & Knoop, C.-I. (2018). Compassionate Management of Mental Health in the Modern Workplace (1st ed. 2018.). Springer International Publishing. https://doi.org/10.1007/978-3-319-71541-4

www.ingramcontent.com/pod-product-compliance
Lightning Source LLC
Chambersburg PA
CBHW030853270326
41928CB00008B/1360